CARDIO
BALL
— FITNESS WORKOUT —

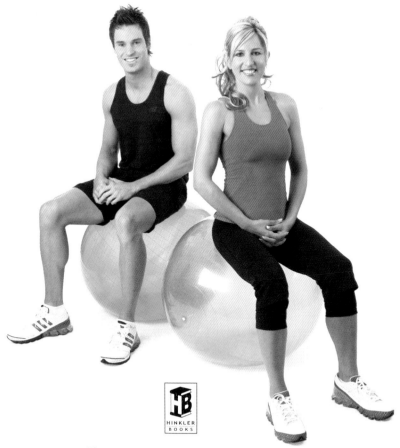

HB
HINKLER
BOOKS

JULIA FILEP

Whether they realise it or not, these people have been instrumental in the creation of Cardio Ball. Words cannot express how much the unconditional friendship, honesty, love, loyalty, motivation, inspiration, and the therapeutic "let's meet for coffee" sessions have meant to me during the writing of this book, and always.

My family: Zoltan, Jacob, Connor, Mum, Dad, Alex, Linda, Alexander, Kane, Anya, Apa, Monika, and Tyler.

Friends and associates: Helen Cuell, the Morey family, the Popovic family, Rod Wilde, Rosemary Nagtegaal, and Rosemary Santos.

You all deserve this public recognition.

"We are more of who we are because of the connections we have made." Adéle Basheer

Julia Filep

Author: Julia Filep
Editors: Katie Hewat and Louise Coulthard
Art Director: Paul Scott
Photography: Ned Meldrum
Prepress: Graphic Print Group

Thanks to Albert Park Yacht Club

First published in 2008
by Hinkler Books Pty Ltd
45–55 Fairchild Street
Heatherton Victoria 3202 Australia
www.hinklerbooks.com

© Hinkler Books Pty Ltd 2008

Printed and bound in China

4 6 8 10 9 7 5 3
09 11 13 12 10

ISBN 978 1 7418 1939 7

CONTENTS

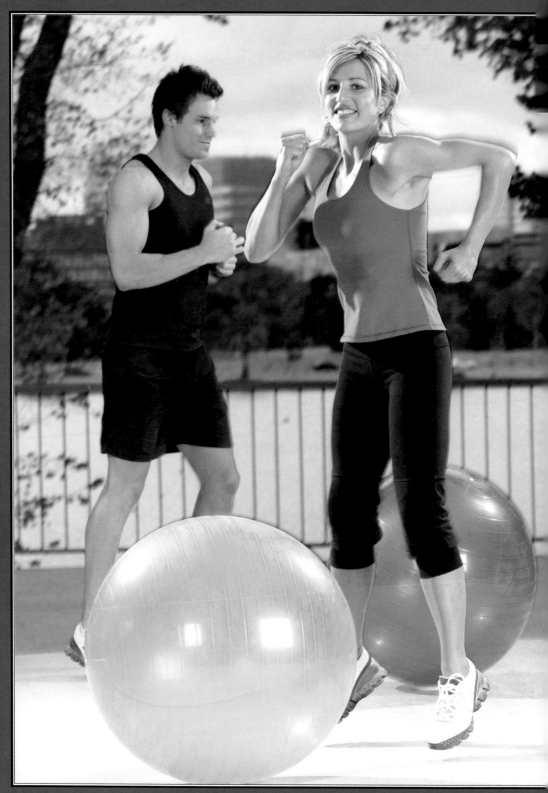

INTRODUCTION

This cardio workout is an easy-to-follow exercise program that addresses the four main aspects of physical fitness.

CARDIO RESPIRATORY ENDURANCE

How efficiently the oxygen and nutrients needed for everyday activity are transported around the body.

MUSCULAR STRENGTH

The greatest amount of force a muscle can exert in a single effort.

MUSCULAR ENDURANCE

The ability of a muscle to repeatedly perform a movement with force for extended periods of time.

FLEXIBILITY

The ability to move a joint through the normal range of motion.

Improving cardio respiratory endurance, muscular strength and muscular endurance has a positive impact on body composition and results in less body fat. Excessive body fat affects physical fitness, reduces the body's performance and negatively affects one's health.

Factors such as speed, agility, muscle power, eye-hand coordination and eye-foot coordination are classified as elements of 'motor' fitness. Appropriate training can improve these factors, leading to a fitter, stronger and more vibrant you!

BEFORE YOU BEGIN

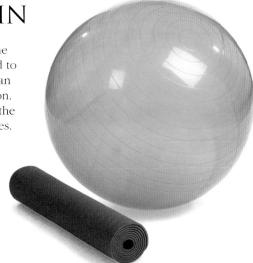

Before you begin the workout, make sure the ball is inflated correctly. It should be inflated to a height so that your bottom is not lower than your knees when you are in a seated position. Otherwise, you can put too much strain on the knee joints and the quadricep (thigh) muscles.

A mat provides necessary padding on the floor while you exercise. A yoga mat (or something similar) is ideal to use during the workout, especially during kneeling, lying and seated exercises.

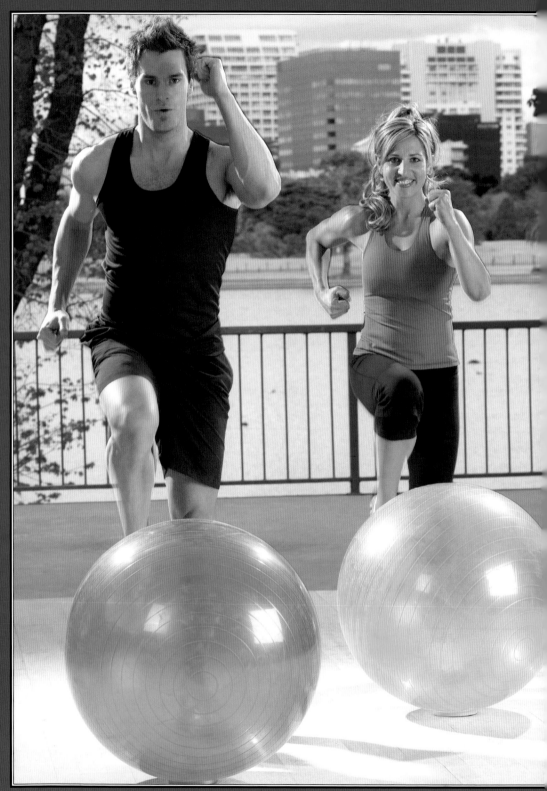

STANDING WARM-UP

The warm-up is the preparation phase of the workout. There are two benefits to the warm-up:

PHYSICAL PREPARATION

Gets blood flowing to all of the major muscles in order to achieve a safe, balanced workout.

MENTAL PREPARATION

Psychologically motivates you to continue with the workout and achieve your goals.

Repeat every exercise in the standing warm-up 10–20 times on each side of the body.

STANDING MASSAGE

Obliques

1 Begin with feet hip-width apart, holding the ball in front of the navel.

2 Swivelling from the hips, twist the torso to the left. Allow the right heel to elevate and the head and neck to follow.

3 Swivel back to the front.

4 Swivelling from the hips, twist the torso to the right side. Allow the left heel to elevate and the head and neck to follow.

5 Continue twisting from one side to the other in a smooth motion.

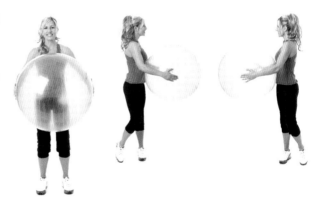

INCREASE THE CHALLENGE

Begin with feet at least shoulder-width apart.

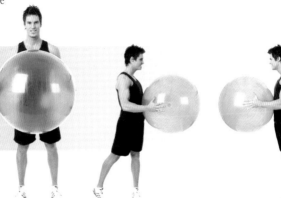

AROUND THE WORLD

Deltoids

1 Begin with feet hip-width apart, holding the ball in front of the navel.

2 Keeping the elbows bent, draw a large circle with the ball by swinging it to the left, then up and over the head and down to the right. Finish back in front of the navel.

3 Repeat on the other side. Continue circling until the shoulders have warmed up.

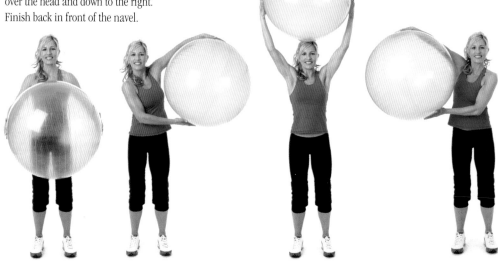

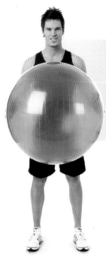

INCREASE THE CHALLENGE

Begin with feet at least shoulder-width apart.

MILITARY MARCHING

Quadriceps

1 Place the ball in front of you on the floor.

2 With a relaxed gait, march on the spot. Keep the shoulders relaxed and lengthen the neck.

3 Maintain a natural easy swinging motion with the arms and brace the core as you march.

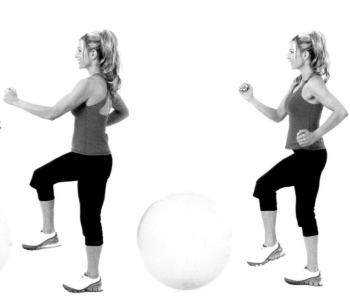

INCREASE THE CHALLENGE

Use a strong swinging motion with the arms as you march.

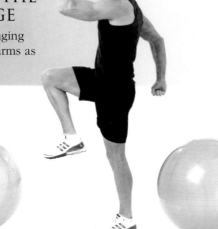

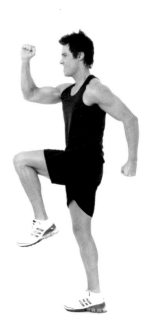

MARCHING AROUND THE WORLD

Hip flexors and quadriceps

1 Place the ball in front of you on the floor. Begin marching on the spot with arms bent like a sprinter.

2 March around the ball in a clockwise direction, making a small circle.

3 Finish behind the ball in the starting position and continue marching on the spot.

4 Repeat, making a circle in the other direction. Don't go too fast around the ball, as it can cause dizziness.

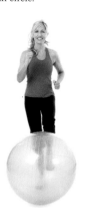 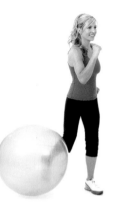 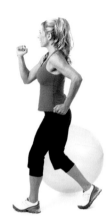 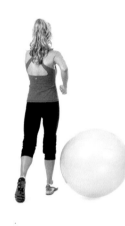

INCREASE THE CHALLENGE

March in large circles around the ball.

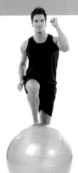 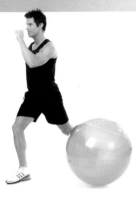 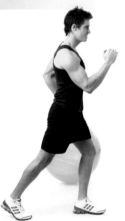 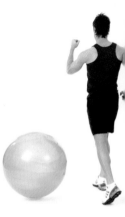

STATUE TAPS

Abdominals and gluteals

1 Place the ball in front of you on the floor. Standing with hands on hips and feet hip-width apart, brace the core muscles.

2 Bend the right knee upwards to elevate the leg.

3 Maintaining your balance, lightly tap the side of the ball with the right toes.

4 Return to the standing position. Repeat with the left leg.

5 Keep alternating the legs while maintaining a tall, upright posture.

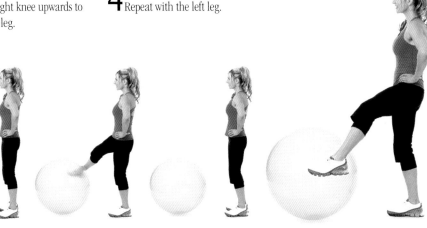

INCREASE THE CHALLENGE

Tap the top of the ball with the toes and swing the arms.

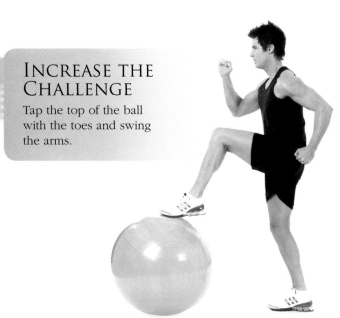

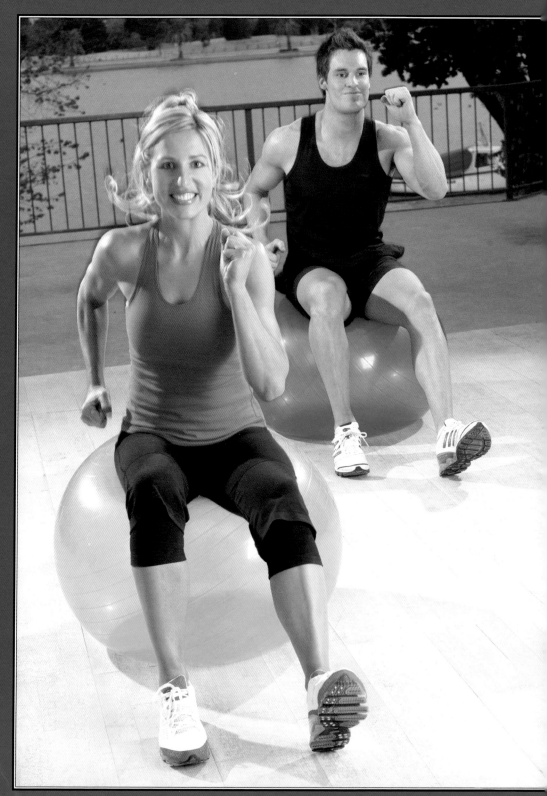

SEATED WARM-UP

Repeat every exercise in the seated warm-up 10–20 times on each side of the body.

REBOUND WITH TOES UP

Abdominals, quadriceps and tibia

1 Start in the seated position with knees at right angles above the ankles. Place hands on hips with the shoulders drawn down.

2 Begin bouncing lightly on the ball with the feet hip-width apart.

3 As you bounce, lift the toes up, keeping both heels 'glued' to the floor. Keep the eyes looking forward.

4 Bounce for 10–20 repetitions or until you feel your heart rate elevate and you are able to maintain the intensity.

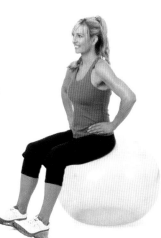
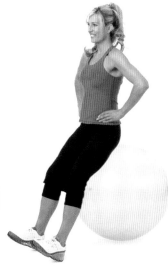
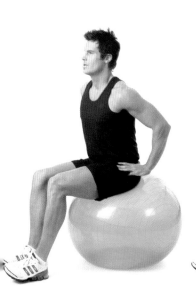
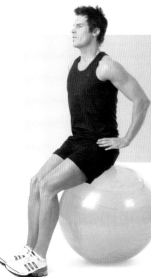

INCREASE THE CHALLENGE

Begin with feet less than hip-width apart to decrease the centre of balance.

REBOUND WITH TOES DOWN

Abdominals, quadriceps and calves

1 Start in the seated position with knees at right angles above the ankles. Place hands on hips with the shoulders drawn down.

2 Begin bouncing lightly on the ball with the feet hip-width apart.

3 As you bounce, lift the heels up, keeping both sets of toes 'glued' to the floor. Keep the eyes looking forward.

4 Bounce for 10–20 repetitions or until you feel your heart rate elevate and you are able to maintain the intensity.

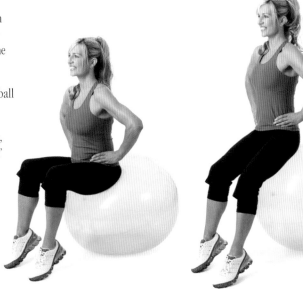

INCREASE THE CHALLENGE

Begin with feet less than hip-width apart to decrease the centre of balance.

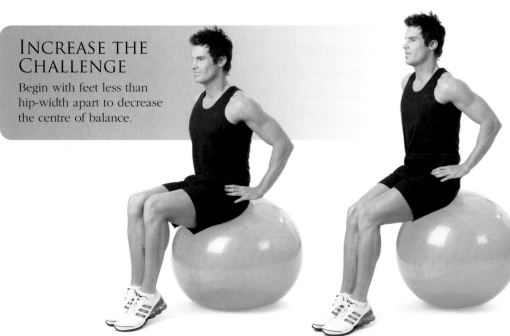

REBOUND DIGGER

Abdominals, quadriceps, calves and tibia

1 Start in the seated position with feet hip-width apart and begin bouncing gently on the ball, swinging the arms.

2 Dig the left heel into the floor as you take a bounce.

3 Bring the right heel back to the starting position on the next bounce.

4 Dig the right heel into the floor with the next bounce.

5 Return the left heel back to the starting position on the following bounce.

6 Continue to alternate the heels for 10–20 repetitions on each side.

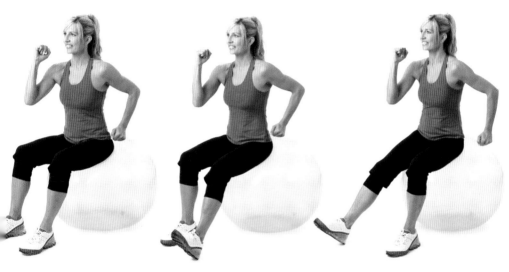

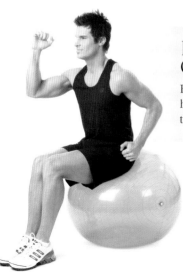

INCREASE THE CHALLENGE

Begin with feet less than hip-width apart to decrease the centre of balance.

RAILWAY REBOUND

Abdominals and quadriceps

1 Begin in the seated position with the arms bent naturally.

2 Keep the knees at right angles above the ankles with the feet hip-width apart.

3 Start bouncing and ensure that the toes are facing forward in a parallel position. Swing the arms in an easy natural motion.

4 When you feel confident, bounce higher off the ball.

5 Bounce for 10–20 repetitions or until you feel your heart rate elevate and you are able to maintain the intensity.

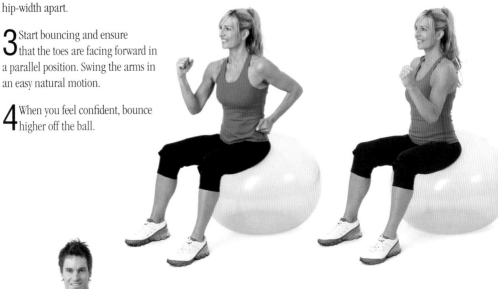

INCREASE THE CHALLENGE

Begin with feet less than hip-width apart to decrease the centre of balance. Swing the arms with a stronger motion.

REBOUND ON OPEN TRACKS

Abdominals, quadriceps and adductors

1 Begin in the seated position with the arms bent naturally.

2 Step both feet out wide with the toes out at a 45-degree angle

3 Start bouncing, ensuring that the toes remain at a 45-degree angle. Keep the knees open, tracking in line with the toes. Swing the arms in an easy natural motion.

4 When you feel confident, bounce higher off the ball.

5 Bounce for 10–20 repetitions or until you feel your heart rate elevate and you are able to maintain the intensity.

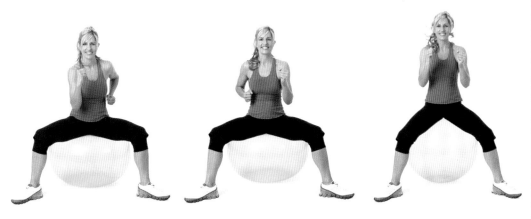

INCREASE THE CHALLENGE
Use a stronger swinging motion with the arms and increase the height of the bounces.

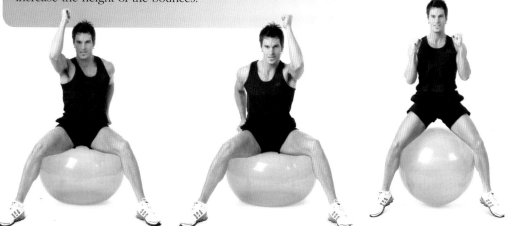

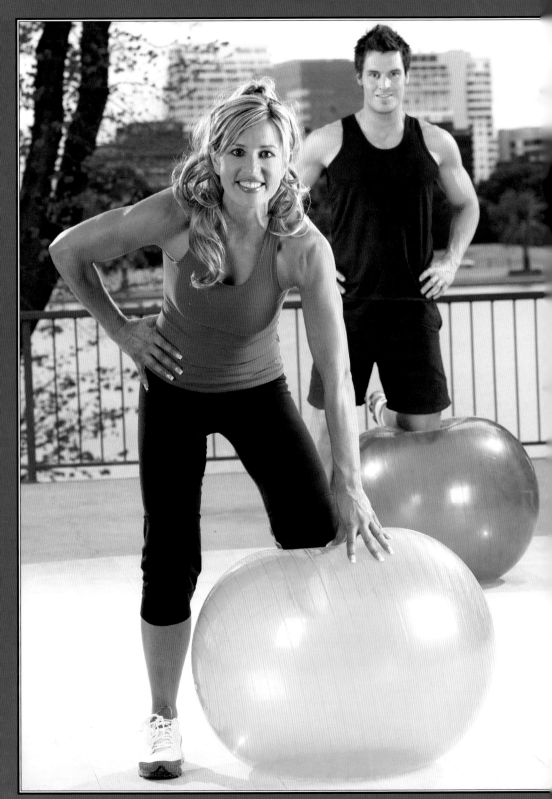

BALANCE

The balance section is a challenging component of this workout. Developing balance skills improves both the body's reaction time and its motor planning. Reaction time is important in many sports and in day-to-day activities.

SEATED MASSAGE (LEFT TO RIGHT)

Abdominals, lower back and pelvis

1 Start in the seated position with knees at right angles above the ankles with the feet hip-width apart. Place hands on hips with the shoulders drawn down.

2 Tip the right hip down slowly and allow the left hip and buttock to lift up and out to the side.

3 Repeat with the left hip and continue, gently rocking side to side.

4 Perform 10–20 repetitions or until you feel the oblique muscles and pelvic area warming up.

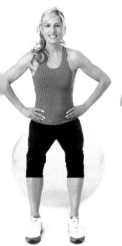 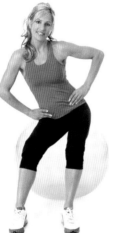 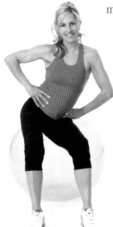

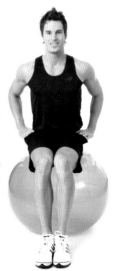

INCREASE THE CHALLENGE

Begin with feet less than hip-width apart to decrease the centre of balance.

BALANCE *(continued)*

SEATED MASSAGE (FORWARD AND BACK)

Abdominals, lower back and pelvis

1 Start in the seated position with knees at right angles above the ankles with the feet hip-width apart. Place hands on hips with the shoulders drawn down.

2 Press down with the hips and tip the pelvis down and forward, making the ball roll backwards a short distance.

3 Reverse this movement and tip the pelvis down and backwards, making the ball roll forward a short distance.

4 Perform 10–20 repetitions or until you feel the abdominal muscles and pelvic area warming up.

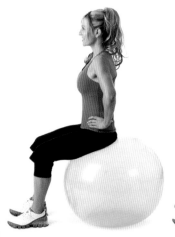 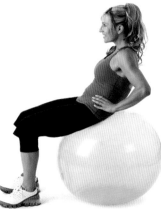 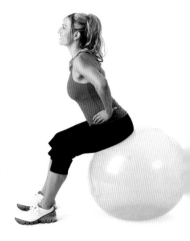

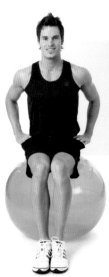

INCREASE THE CHALLENGE

Begin with feet less than hip-width apart to decrease the centre of balance.

THE CRANE

Abdominals, lower back, pelvis and quadriceps

1 Start in the seated position with knees at right angles above the ankles with the feet hip-width apart. Place hands on hips with the shoulders drawn down. Remain stationary on the ball.

2 Elevate the right foot off the floor slightly and try to maintain your balance.

3 Hold this position for as long as possible. Use the arms to help with balance if necessary.

4 Repeat with the left foot.

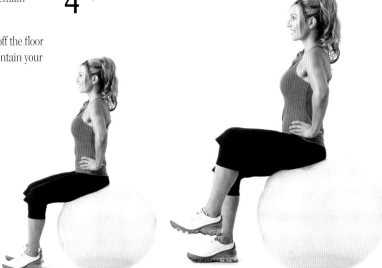

INCREASE THE CHALLENGE

Begin with feet less than hip-width apart to decrease the centre of balance, and elevate the foot higher off the floor.

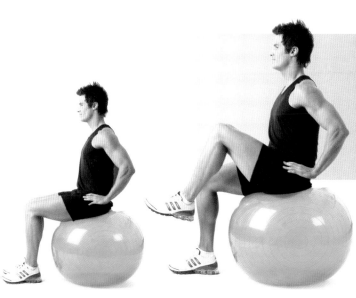

BALANCE *(continued)*

ONE-LEGGED STATUE

Abdominals, lower back, pelvis and quadriceps

1 Stand with the ball next to you on the left.

2 Carefully lean sideways and place both hands on the ball, followed by the left knee.

3 While the right leg remains on the floor, negotiate your balance by applying weight to the standing right leg and then to the left knee.

4 When confident, let go with one hand, using the arms to assist with balance. This requires plenty of practice. Balance for as long as possible.

5 Repeat with the right leg.

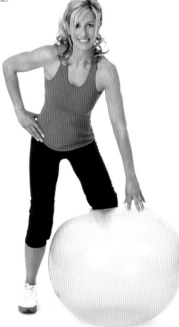

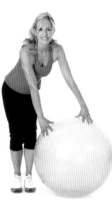

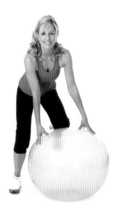

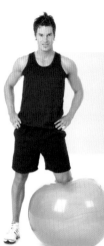

INCREASE THE CHALLENGE

Take both hands off the ball.

THE BALANCING STATUE

Abdominals, lower back, pelvis, quadriceps and tibia

1 Place the ball against a wall and stand on the other side, resting one hand on the wall and the other hand on the ball.

2 Using the leg closest to the wall, kneel on the ball while keeping your hand on it.

3 Slowly transfer your weight on to the ball, and then kneel on the ball with the other knee.

4 Keeping one hand on the wall, kneel upright on the ball with knees wide apart. Anchor the toes into the ball to stabilise yourself and do not sit on your heels. Balance on the ball for as long as possible. This requires plenty of practice.

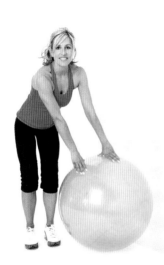 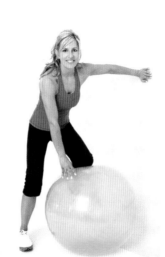 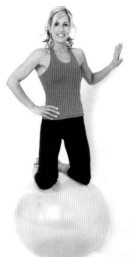

INCREASE THE CHALLENGE

Take both hands off the wall and place them on your hips.

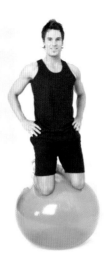

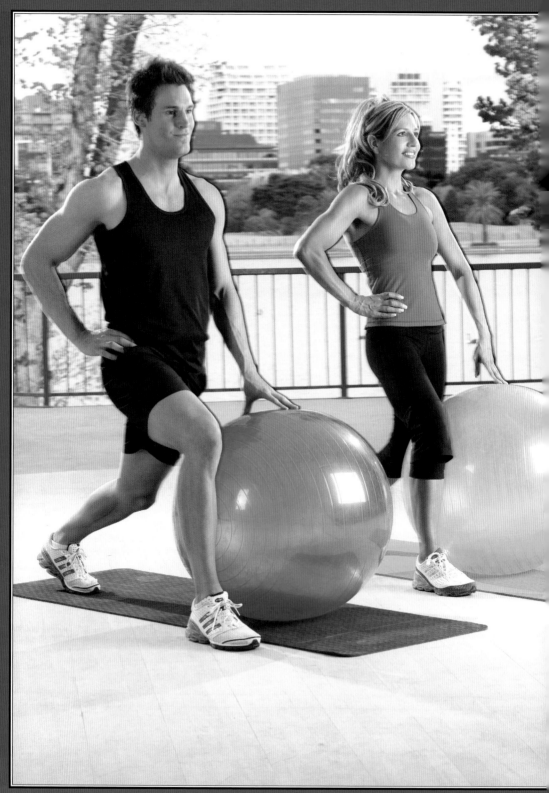

DYNAMIC STRETCHES

Dynamic movements are the best way to prepare your body for dynamic workouts. This involves taking the muscle to a repeated elongated position with gentle recovery. Dynamic stretches are best done after a warm-up routine. A static stretch is a stationary or fixed stretch. Contrary to old beliefs, the best time to work on static stretching is at the end of the workout, not at the beginning.

Repeat dynamic stretches 4 times on each side of the body and hold each dynamic stretch for 2–4 counts.

SPIDER STRETCH

Abdominals and adductors

1 Begin in the seated position with hands on hips.

2 Step the feet out wider than the shoulders with the toes facing forward.

3 Maintaining an upright posture, lean over to the right. Allow the ball to roll to the left underneath your bottom as you bend the right knee and straighten the left leg.

4 Hold the stretch for 4 counts and then repeat to the left.

5 Complete this sequence on each side 4 times.

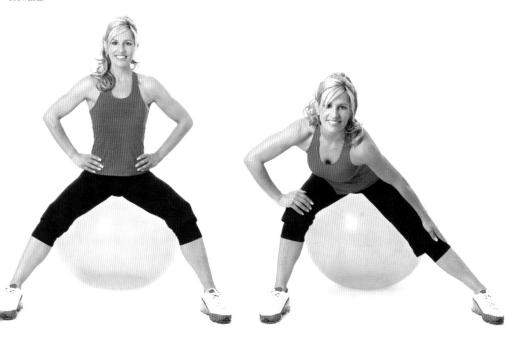

DYNAMIC STRETCHES *(continued)*

SEATED SCISSOR STRETCH

Abdominals and hamstrings

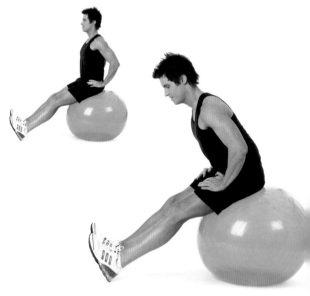

1 Begin in the seated position with hands on hips.

2 Place both heels forward on the floor hip-width apart.

3 Gently tip forward from the hips without slouching. Rest the hands on the thighs (not the knees) or further down if your flexibility allows.

4 Hold this stretch for 4 counts and then move back into an upright seated position.

5 Complete this sequence 4 times.

STANDING TUCK

Hip flexors

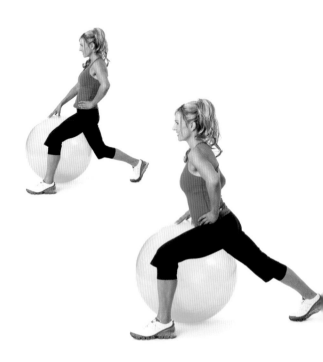

1 Stand behind the ball with the feet hip-width apart and the toes facing forward.

2 Step back with the right foot, maintaining the feet in a parallel position to open the hip joint.

3 Hug the ball into the open hip and lift the back heel off the floor.

4 Using a gentle rhythmic action, tilt the pelvis forward and then back 8 times.

5 Repeat this sequence with the other leg.

WALL PUSH

Calves

1 Place the ball against a wall and stand behind the ball with feet hip-width apart.

2 Lean forward and place both hands on the ball, keeping them shoulder-width apart.

3 Extend one leg back and press the heel into the floor while pushing the other bent knee into the ball.

4 Using a gentle rhythmic action, lift and then press the heel into the floor 8 times.

5 Repeat with the other leg.

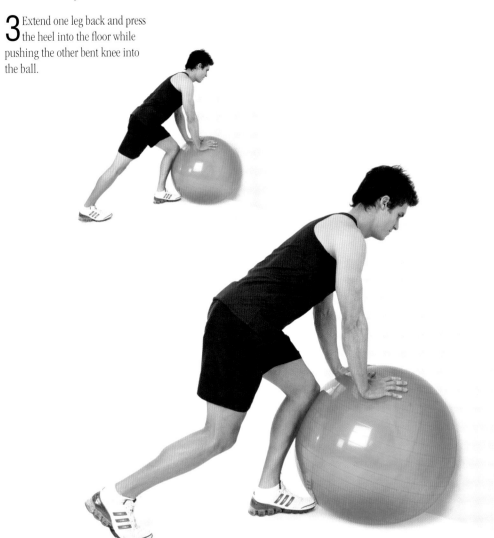

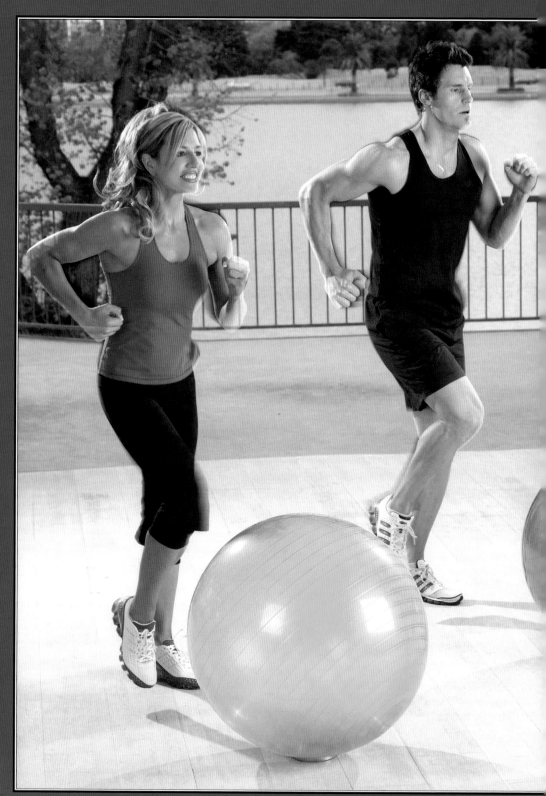

STANDING CARDIO

This is the fitness component of the workout. Cardio exercise challenges the heart and lungs. It improves your respiratory efficiency, which means how efficiently the heart, blood vessels and lungs deliver oxygen to the muscles and remove waste products.

Repeat each standing cardio exercise 16 times on each side of the body, then 8 times and then 4 times.

KNEE JAM

Abdominals, hip flexors and quadriceps

1 Stand with the feet hip-width apart and hold the ball in front of your chest.

2 Elevate the left leg off the floor, bending the knee to hip level. At the same time, lower the ball down in front of you so it touches the left knee.

3 Lower the left leg back to the standing position while lifting the ball back to chest height. Ensure the abdominals remain braced and the eyes are looking to the front.

4 Repeat with the right leg.

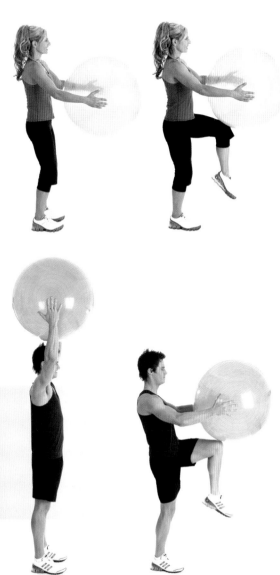

INCREASE THE CHALLENGE

Start by holding the ball above the head instead of in front of the chest and return the ball to head height after each repetition.

SHUFFLE AROUND THE WORLD

Abductors, gluteals, ankles and calves

1 Place the ball on the floor in front of you. Wait for the ball to come to a complete rest, then bend the arms like a sprinter.

2 Stand with your feet hip-width apart. Begin bouncing on the balls of the feet, allowing the arms to pump with each bounce.

3 Keeping the hips facing the ball, bounce around the ball to the left in a continuous motion until you have done a complete circle and are back where you started.

4 Repeat, bouncing to the right side in a continuous motion until you have done a complete circle and are back where you started.

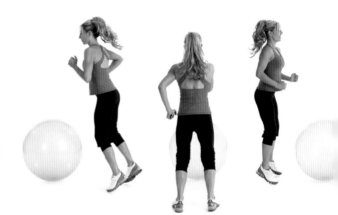

INCREASE THE CHALLENGE

Stand with your feet shoulder-width apart and make a larger circle around the ball so that you travel further. Pump the arms more vigorously as you circle.

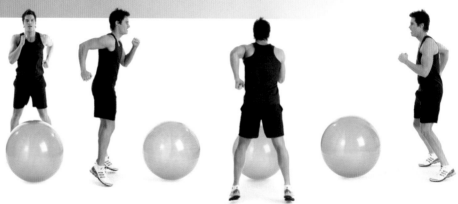

SPRINTS

Quadriceps and calves

1 Stand behind the ball with the feet hip-width apart. Bend both arms like a sprinter.

2 Begin a light jog on the spot using short, rapid foot strikes.

3 Alternate the arms to build up the intensity.

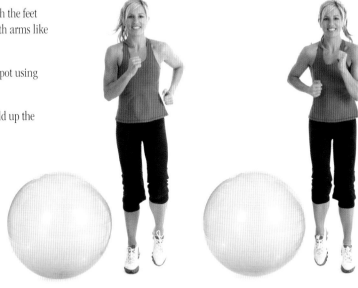

INCREASE THE CHALLENGE

Start with a heavy jog and use high, rapid foot strikes.

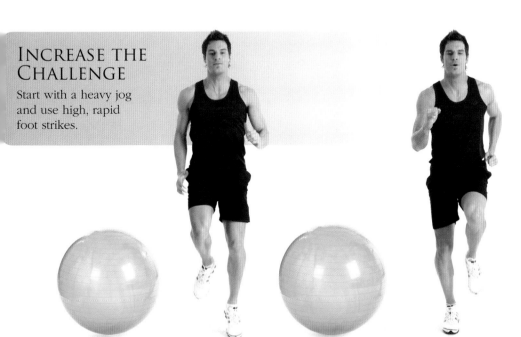

STANDING CARDIO *(continued)*

THE PUNCHING BAG

Biceps, deltoids and pectorals

1 Place the ball on the floor against a wall. Prop the left knee on the ball and apply pressure to keep it firmly against the wall.

2 Make a fist with both hands, ensuring both thumbs are on the outside.

3 Punch the ball with slow, alternating strikes, keeping the elbows close to the sides of the torso and bracing the core muscles.

4 Gradually build up the speed of the strikes.

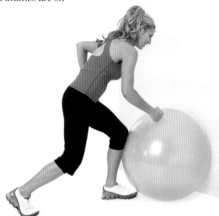 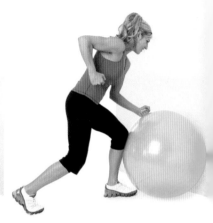

INCREASE THE CHALLENGE

Punch the ball with fast, alternating strikes.

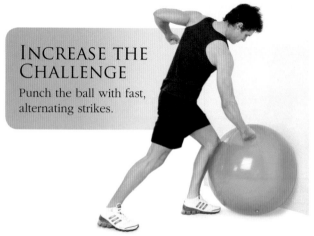 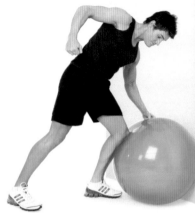

SCISSORS

Quadriceps and calves

1 Place the ball on the floor against a wall. Lean forward and place both hands on the ball as a base of support.

2 Keeping the hands on the ball, shoulder-width apart, begin slowly shuffling the feet forward and back in a scissor-like action. Ensure the feet remain parallel and the toes face forward.

3 Maintain the same speed with each alternating heel strike.

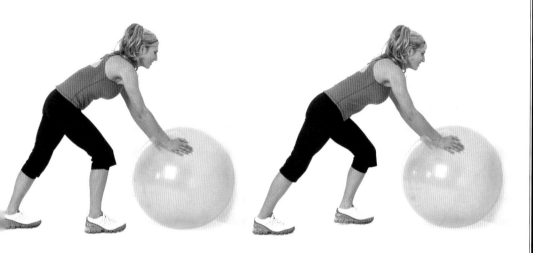

INCREASE THE CHALLENGE

Begin by shuffling the feet forward and back at a faster speed, while keeping the heels off the ground.

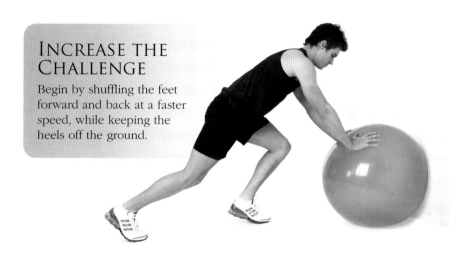

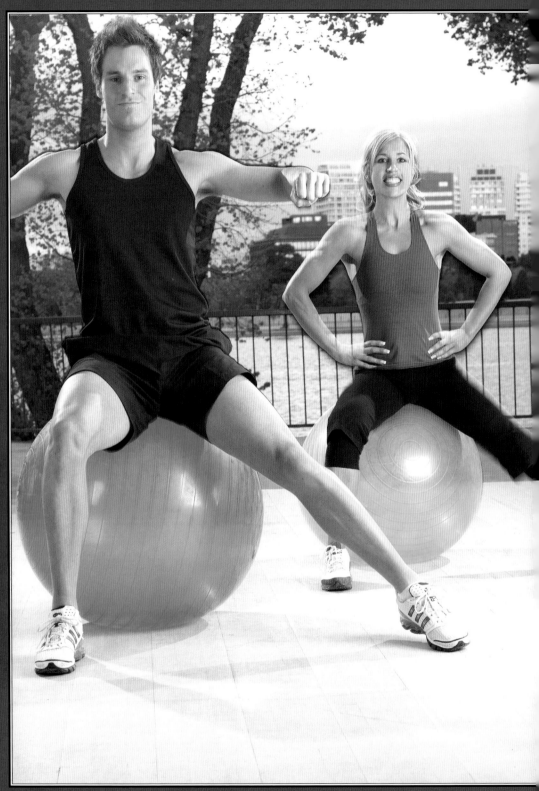

SEATED CARDIO

Repeat each seated cardio exercise 16 times on each side of the body, then 8 times and then 4 times.

REBOUND TAP

Abdominals, adductors, quadriceps and deltoids

1 Bounce lightly in the seated position with your feet hip-width apart and hands on hips.

2 On the first bounce, tap the right foot on the floor out to the right.

3 Bring the right foot back to the starting position on the second bounce.

4 On the third bounce, tap the left foot on the floor out to the left.

5 Bring the left foot back to the starting position on the next bounce.

6 Continue to bounce and tap while lifting the arms to the side with bent elbows for more intensity.

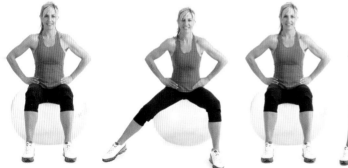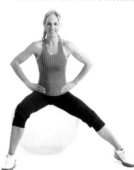

INCREASE THE CHALLENGE

Begin with feet less than hip-width apart to decrease the centre of balance.

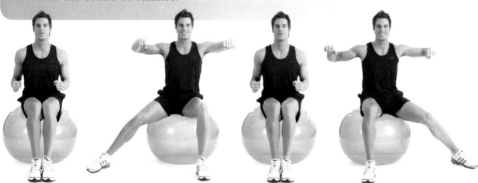

REBOUND JACK

Abdominals, adductors and quadriceps

1 Bounce lightly in the seated position with your feet on the floor hip-width apart.

2 Jump both feet out wide on the floor with the first bounce.

3 Bring both feet back to hip-width on the floor with the second bounce.

4 Once a rhythm is established, incorporate both of the arms by lifting them to the side with bent elbows for more intensity.

5 On the first bounce when the feet jump out wide, lift both arms to the side with the elbows bent.

6 On the second bounce when the feet jump back to the middle, lower both arms down beside the body with the elbows bent.

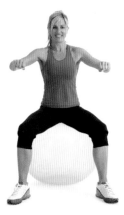
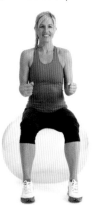
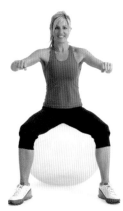

INCREASE THE CHALLENGE

Begin with feet touching together on the floor to decrease the centre of balance.

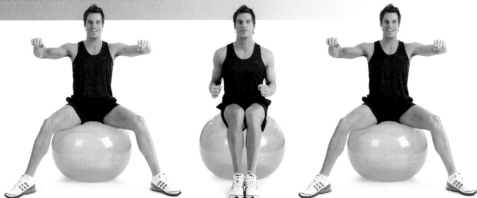

GUM BOOT MARCHING

Abdominals and quadriceps

1 Begin in the seated position on the ball, with hands on hips. Bounce on the ball, looking straight ahead.

2 With each bounce, alternately elevate each foot off the floor a little, as though you are marching. Imagine you have big boots on your feet as you march.

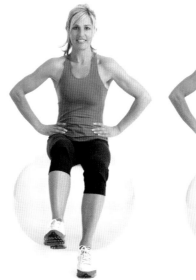
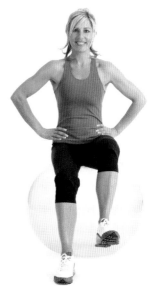

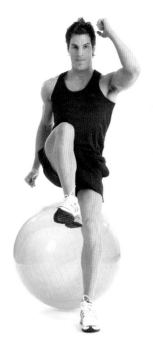
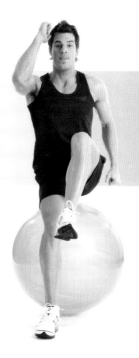

INCREASE THE CHALLENGE

Swing the arms and elevate the feet higher as you march.

GUM BOOT HOP

Abdominals, adductors and quadriceps

1 Begin in the seated position on the ball, with hands on hips. Bounce on the ball, looking straight ahead.

2 With each bounce, alternately elevate each foot off the floor a little, as though you are marching.

3 Replace the single bounce with a double bounce. This is more challenging for your balance.

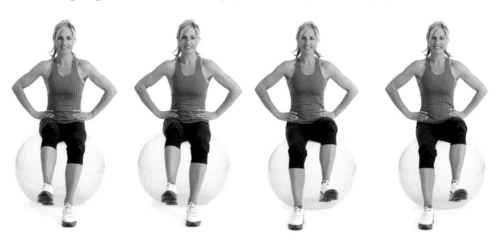

INCREASE THE CHALLENGE

Swing the arms and elevate the feet higher as you march.

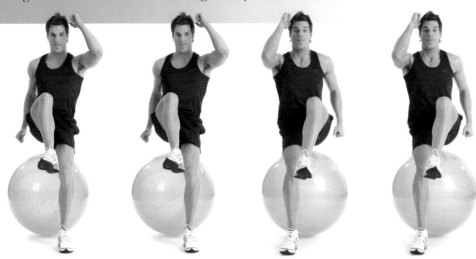

REBOUND

Abdominals, gluteals and quadriceps

1 Begin in the seated position on the ball. Bounce on the ball, looking straight ahead. Rest your hands beside you on the ball.

2 Bounce four times and then lift the buttocks off the ball. Support yourself by resting one hand on the ball. Reach the other hand out. Pause for a moment with the buttocks off the ball between each bouncing sequence.

3 Continue the sequence, bouncing three times and then lifting the buttocks off the ball. Pause and reach the hand out.

4 Continue the sequence and bounce two times and then lift the buttocks off the ball. Pause and reach the hand out.

5 Continue the sequence and bounce once and then lift the buttocks off the ball. Pause and reach the hand out.

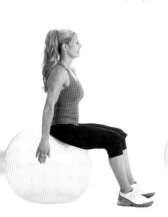
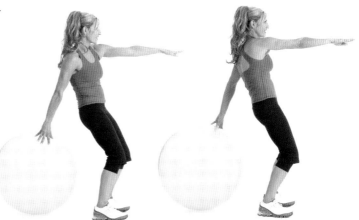

INCREASE THE CHALLENGE

Begin with feet less than hip-width apart to decrease the centre of balance.

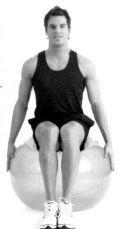

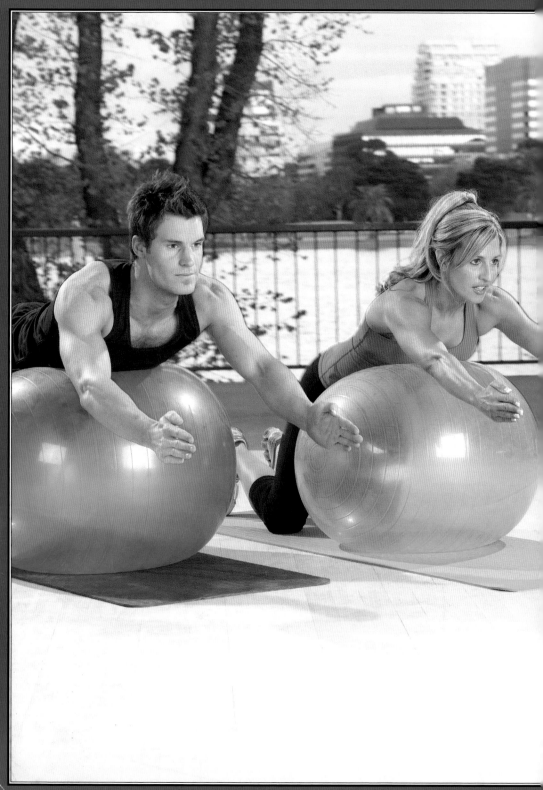

MUSCLE CONDITIONING

Muscle strength and endurance are two of the four components of physical fitness (see page 5). The following exercises will help improve functional strength and endurance for everyday 'incidental' activities, such as gardening, walking up stairs, lifting and carrying objects, and housework.

Repeat 3 sets of each muscle conditioning exercise, with 10–15 repetitions of each exercise in each set.

LUNGES WITH BALL IN FRONT

Quadriceps, gluteals and calves

1 Stand beside the ball with the feet hip-width apart and toes parallel.

2 Resting your hand on the ball for balance, take a long step forward and keep the front knee in line above the ankle.

3 Lift the back heel off the floor and tuck the pelvis under.

4 Bend the rear leg and lower the body halfway down with both knees. Maintain good posture, keeping the shoulders in a vertical line above the hips. Repeat with the same leg 10–15 times.

5 Push off with the front foot back to the standing position.

6 Repeat the sequence with the other leg 10–15 times.

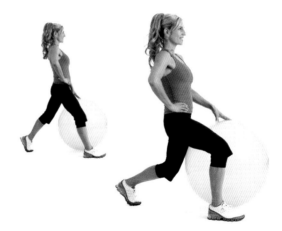

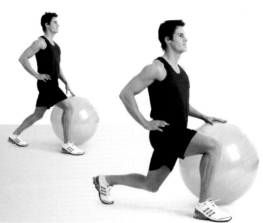

INCREASE THE CHALLENGE
Lower the body down to a right angle.

MUSCLE CONDITIONING *(continued)*

LUNGES WITH BALL BEHIND

Quadriceps, gluteals and calves

1 Position the ball against a wall between your mid and lower spine. Keep your back upright and place hands on hips.

2 Take a long step forward and keep the front knee bent in line above the ankle.

3 Lift the back heel off the floor and tuck the pelvis under.

4 Bend the rear leg and lower the body halfway down with both knees. Maintain good posture with the shoulders in a vertical line above the hips. Repeat with the same leg 10–15 times.

5 Push off with the front foot back to the standing position.

6 Repeat the sequence with the other leg 10–15 times.

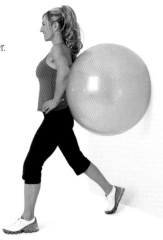 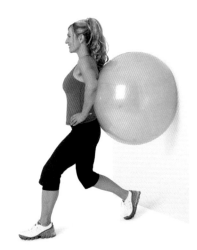

INCREASE THE CHALLENGE

Lower the body down to a right angle and pulse in the lowered position 10–15 times.

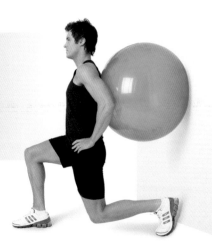

WALKING WHEELBARROW

Abdominals, deltoids, lower back and pectorals

1 Kneel on the floor behind the ball and then roll forward over the ball. Walk your arms forward until your thighs are on the ball. Keep the fingers facing forward and the hands shoulder-width apart.

2 Draw the abdominal muscles up high towards your spine and keep the torso straight like a table. Hold this position for 30 seconds or as long as possible.

3 Walk your arms backward and finish kneeling behind the ball.

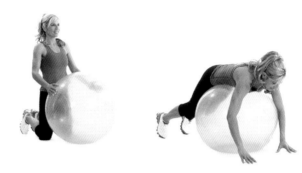

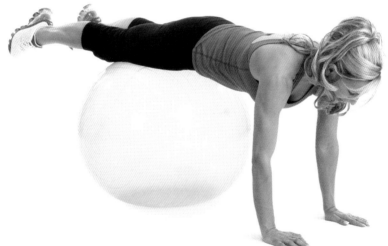

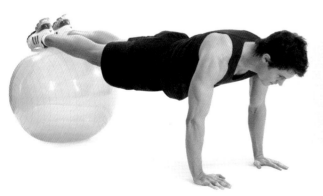

INCREASE THE CHALLENGE

Walk your arms forward until your feet are on the ball.

MUSCLE CONDITIONING *(continued)*

WALKING WHEELBARROWS WITH PUSH-UPS

Abdominals, deltoids, lower back, pectorals and triceps

1 Kneel on the floor behind the ball and then roll forward over the ball. Walk your arms forward until your thighs are on the ball. Keep the fingers facing forward and the hands shoulder-width apart.

2 Draw the abdominal muscles up high towards your spine and keep the torso straight like a table.

3 Bend your elbows, lowering the chest to the floor until your chin nearly touches the floor.

4 Push back up slowly, avoiding locking the elbows at the top.

5 Walk your arms backward and finish kneeling behind the ball.

6 Repeat the exercise 10–15 times, rolling forward, completing push-up and rolling back each time.

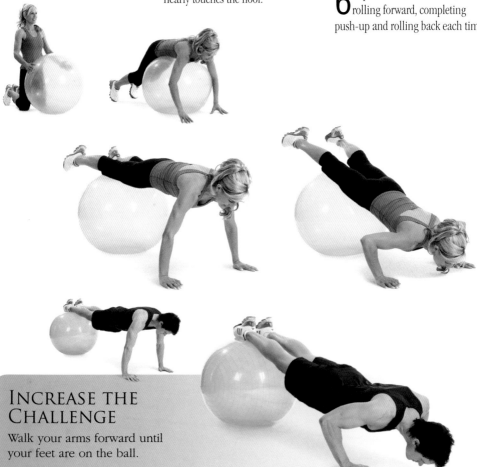

INCREASE THE CHALLENGE

Walk your arms forward until your feet are on the ball.

TRICEP PUSH-UPS

Triceps and pectorals

1 Place the ball on the floor against a wall and kneel about a foot away from it, ensuring that the toes are tucked under the heels to anchor the body.

2 Lean forward and place both hands on the ball no more than shoulder-width apart.

3 Keep palms on the ball, fingers pointing up and elbows pointing to the rear close to the torso.

4 Bend both elbows and lower your chest halfway to the ball.

5 Slowly push up, keeping the elbows tucked in close to the waist. Avoid locking the elbows.

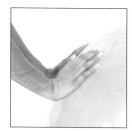

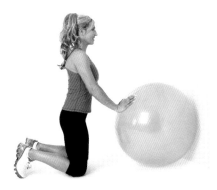

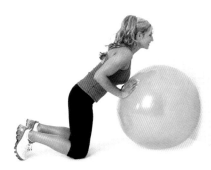

INCREASE THE CHALLENGE

Raise yourself on your toes behind the ball instead of kneeling. Tuck in the tail bone and lower your chest all the way to the ball.

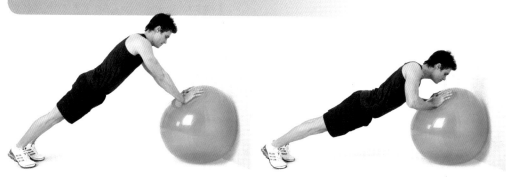

MUSCLE CONDITIONING *(continued)*

BICEP PUSH-UPS

Deltoids, biceps and abdominals

1 Place the ball on the floor against a wall. Kneel with knees hip-width apart about a foot from the ball, ensuring that the toes are tucked under the heels to anchor the body.

2 Lean forward and place both hands on the ball no more than shoulder-width apart.

3 Keep palms on the ball, fingers pointing out and down, elbows pointing to the rear close to the torso.

4 Bend both elbows and lower your chest halfway to the ball.

5 Slowly push up, keeping the elbows tucked in close to the waist. Avoid locking the elbows.

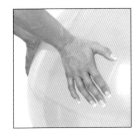

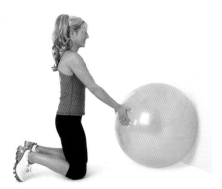

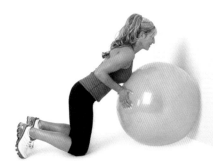

INCREASE THE CHALLENGE

Raise yourself on your toes behind the ball instead of kneeling. Tuck in the tail bone and lower your chest all the way to the ball.

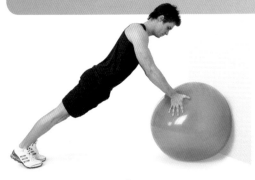

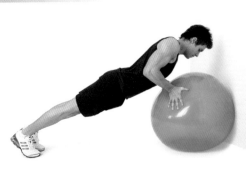

THE SEATED WALKER

Abdominals, gluteals and hamstrings

1 Begin in the seated position with arms crossing the chest, keeping the neck long and looking forward.

2 Walk the feet forward, keeping them hip-width apart. Allow the ball to roll along the spine, keeping the torso strong and stable. Stop walking when the ball is at the upper back.

3 Brace the abdominal wall, keeping the torso straight like a table. Contract the buttocks to hold this position, and pause for a moment.

4 Walk the feet backward, again keeping the torso strong and stable. Allow the ball to roll along the spine.

5 Walk back until you are in the seated position.

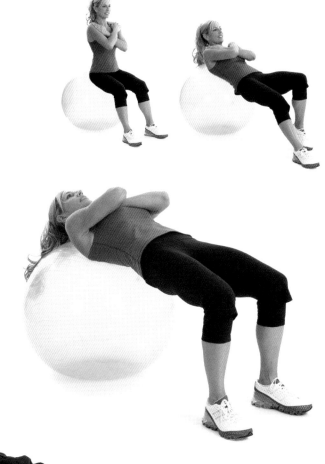

INCREASE THE CHALLENGE

Begin with feet less than hip-width apart to decrease the centre of balance and stop walking when the ball is at the base of the neck.

MUSCLE CONDITIONING (continued)

THE CRUCIFIX

*Abdominals, gluteals,
hamstrings and obliques*

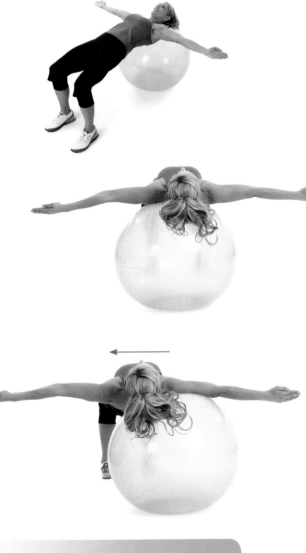

1 Sit on the ball. Walk the feet forward as you lean back on the ball until the shoulders rest on it. Head and neck should be comfortable and knees should be directly above the ankles. Feet should remain hip-width apart. If your chin is on your chest, walk the feet back a little.

2 Open both arms out to the sides in line with the chest and shoulders. To hold this position, press down with the heels and squeeze the buttocks to keep the hips up.

3 Take small, shuffling steps to the side until the ball is off centre under your back. Use the strength in your abdominals and buttocks to keep the body still and parallel with the floor.

4 Hold this position for as long as possible and then repeat to the other side.

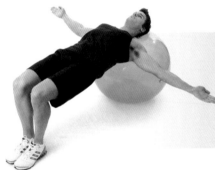

INCREASE THE CHALLENGE

Begin with feet less than hip-width apart to decrease the centre of balance.

THE PLANK

Abdominals, obliques and lower back

1 Kneel on the floor behind the ball and roll forward over it. Walk the arms forward until the thighs are on the ball.

2 Place both elbows on the floor at right angles, directly under the shoulders.

3 Hold this position for 30 seconds or as long as possible.

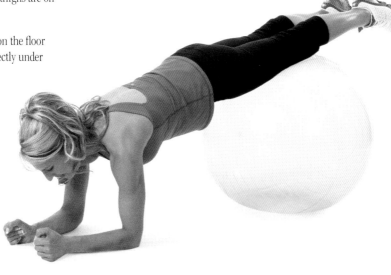

INCREASE THE CHALLENGE

Walk your arms forward until your feet are on the ball.

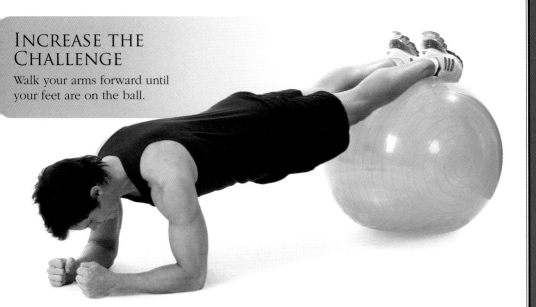

Muscle Conditioning *(continued)*

The Broken Plank

Abdominals, obliques, lower back, deltoids and pectorals

1 Kneel on the floor behind the ball and roll forward over it. Walk the arms forward until the thighs are on the ball.

2 Place both elbows on the floor at right angles, directly under the shoulders.

3 Lift the buttocks and hips into a pike position, drawing the knees up towards the chest.

4 Hold this position and then return to the hover position. Do not allow the abdominals to sag down as this puts pressure on the lower back.

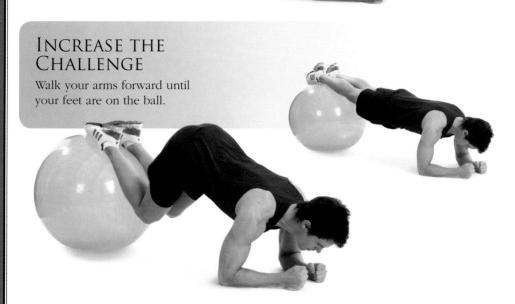

Increase the Challenge

Walk your arms forward until your feet are on the ball.

ROW THE BOAT

Abdominals and lower back

1 Kneel with knees hip-width apart behind the ball. Lean forward so the stomach and hips are on the ball, keeping both knees on the floor.

2 Raise the head, neck and chest off the ball and reach both arms out in front.

3 Pull and reach the arms in a continuous motion, as though you are rowing a boat. Keep the elbows close to the torso and the hips, torso and neck elongated.

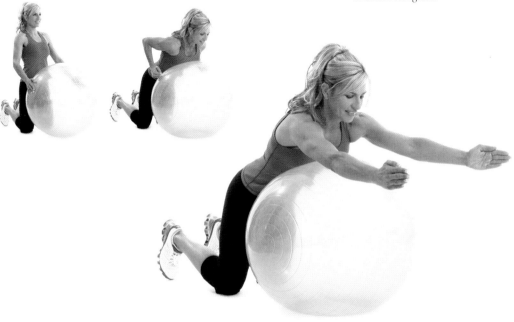

INCREASE THE CHALLENGE

Raise yourself on your toes behind the ball instead of kneeling and keep feet together.

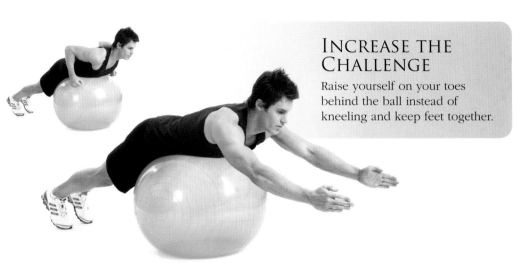

MUSCLE CONDITIONING *(continued)*

THE DRAPE

Upper neck and lower back

1 Kneel with knees hip-width apart behind the ball. Lean forward so the stomach and hips are on the ball.

2 Roll the body forward over the ball and hug it.

3 Allow your entire body to collapse over the ball. Relax and remain in this position for 30 seconds.

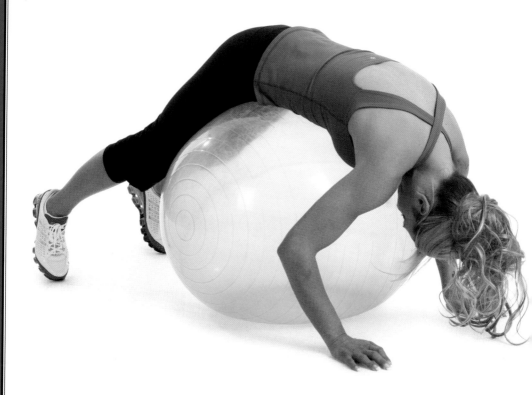

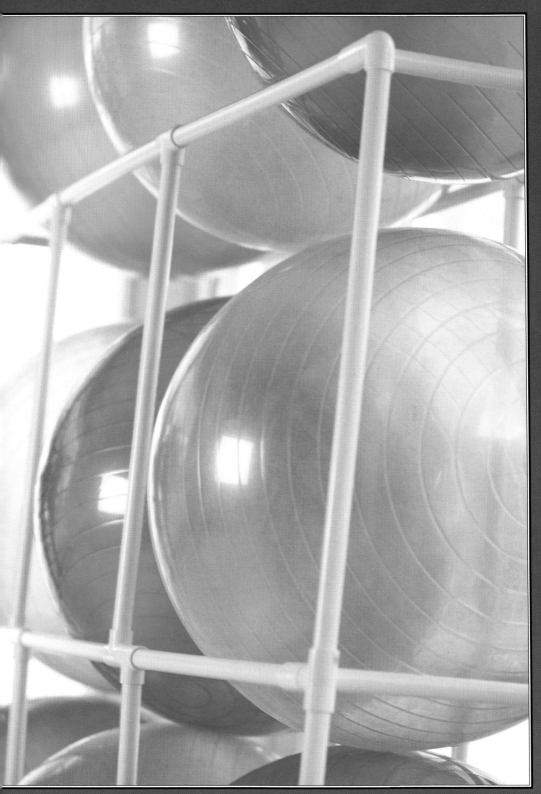

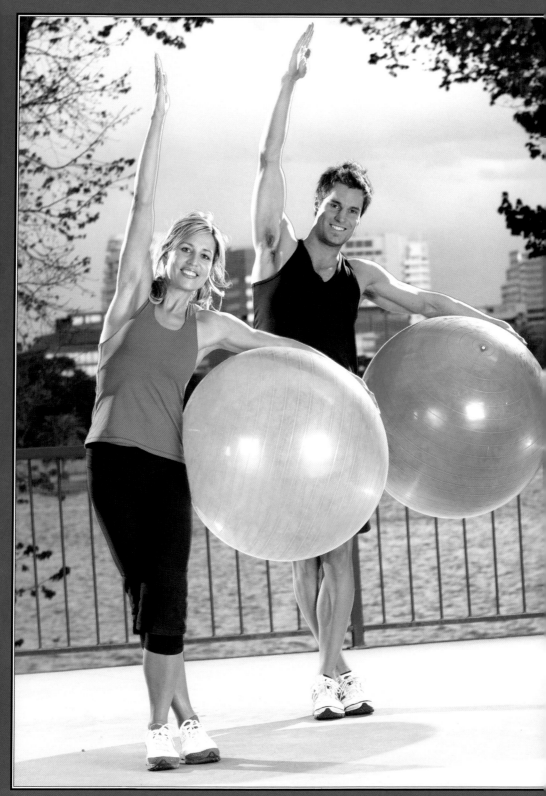

STATIC STRETCHES

Each workout should always be followed by 4–6 minutes of static stretching. Static stretching lengthens a muscle to an elongated position for 20 seconds. Continue to use functional breathing throughout the stretches and avoid holding your breath. Allow this to be the maintenance and reflection part of your workout.

HAMSTRING STRETCH

Hamstrings

1 Lie on your back and rest your calves on the ball.

2 Reach up and cup your hands behind your right knee joint.

3 Gently pull your right leg in towards your body with the knee bent. Keep your lower spine and buttocks in contact with the floor.

4 Hold this stretch for 20 seconds and then repeat with the left leg.

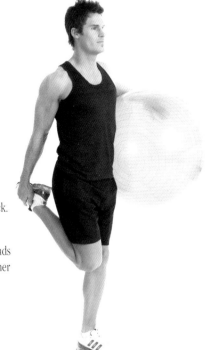

THE STANDING TWEEZER STRETCH

Quadriceps

1 Stand with your feet hip-width apart. Tuck the ball under your left arm.

2 Lift the right foot out behind you and balance carefully on the left leg.

3 Using your right hand, pull your right heel into your right buttock.

4 Imagine you are tweezing together the heel and buttock. Keep your eyes fixed forward.

5 Hold the stretch for 20 seconds and then repeat with the other foot.

STATIC STRETCHES *(continued)*

THE 90/90 STRETCH

Gluteals

1 Sit on the floor on your left buttock. Bend the knees at right angles pointing towards the right side of the body.

2 Place the hands on the floor on either side of the front left leg and tip forward from the hips.

3 Lower the breastbone towards the front left knee.

4 Hold the stretch for 20 seconds and then repeat on the other side, changing sides by swivelling on the tailbone.

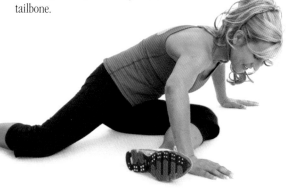

THE WALL TIP STRETCH

Achilles

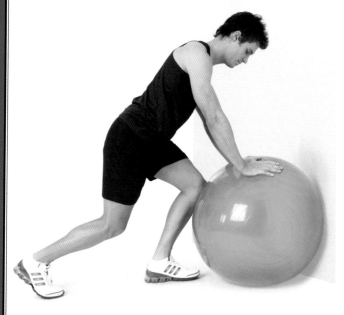

1 Place the ball on the floor against a wall. Prop the left knee on the ball and apply pressure so the ball sits firmly against the wall.

2 Extend the right leg out behind the ball and place the heel on the floor.

3 Bend the knee slightly and lift the heel about an inch off the floor.

4 Hold the stretch for 20 seconds and then repeat with the other foot.

THE WALL PUSH STRETCH

Calves

1 Place the ball on the floor against a wall. Prop the left knee on the ball and apply pressure so the ball sits firmly against the wall. Press both palms into the ball.

2 Extend the left leg out behind the ball and press firmly through the heel into the floor.

3 Hold the stretch for 20 seconds and then repeat with the other foot.

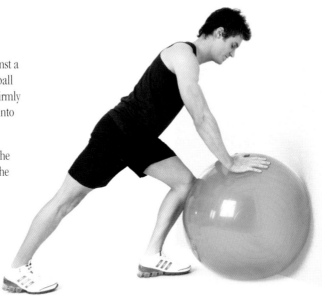

KNEELING TUCK STRETCH

Hip flexors

1 Begin by kneeling on the floor with knees hip-width apart.

2 Take a generous step forward onto the foot with the left leg.

3 Ensure that the front knee is aligned directly above the left ankle.

4 Place both hands onto the top of the left thigh muscle.

5 Gently press forward through the front of the left hip.

6 Hold this stretch for 20 seconds and then repeat with left leg.

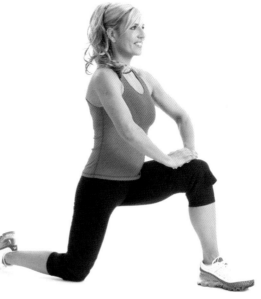

STATIC STRETCHES *(continued)*

I SURRENDER STRETCH

Deltoids, biceps and pectorals

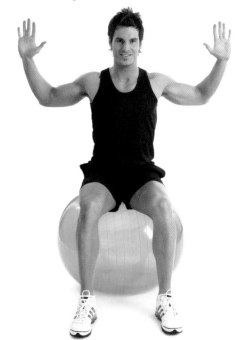

1 Begin in a seated position on the ball, feet hip-width apart.

2 Keep the eyes focused forward, lift the chest and draw the shoulders up and back.

3 Take both of the arms out to the sides at shoulder height.

4 Bend both of the elbows to a right angle with palms open.

5 Squeeze both of the elbows back.

6 Hold this stretch for 20 seconds.

HINGE STRETCH

Triceps

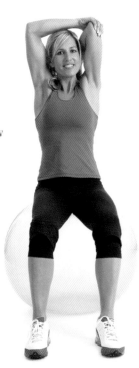

1 Sit upright on the ball, looking straight ahead. Draw in your belly button and raise one arm above the head.

2 Bend the arm backwards at the elbow and reach down the spine with your hand.

3 Place the other hand on the elbow and gently press until you feel a stretch.

4 Hold the stretch for 20 seconds and then repeat with the other arm.

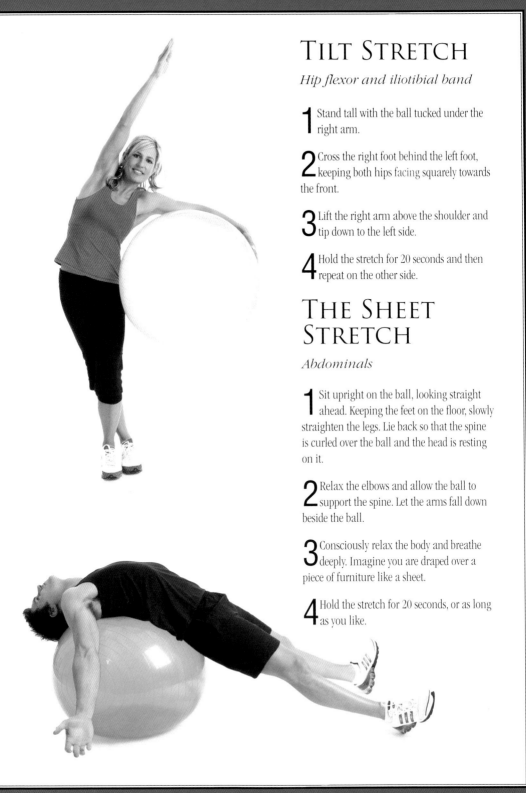

TILT STRETCH

Hip flexor and iliotibial band

1 Stand tall with the ball tucked under the right arm.

2 Cross the right foot behind the left foot, keeping both hips facing squarely towards the front.

3 Lift the right arm above the shoulder and tip down to the left side.

4 Hold the stretch for 20 seconds and then repeat on the other side.

THE SHEET STRETCH

Abdominals

1 Sit upright on the ball, looking straight ahead. Keeping the feet on the floor, slowly straighten the legs. Lie back so that the spine is curled over the ball and the head is resting on it.

2 Relax the elbows and allow the ball to support the spine. Let the arms fall down beside the ball.

3 Consciously relax the body and breathe deeply. Imagine you are draped over a piece of furniture like a sheet.

4 Hold the stretch for 20 seconds, or as long as you like.

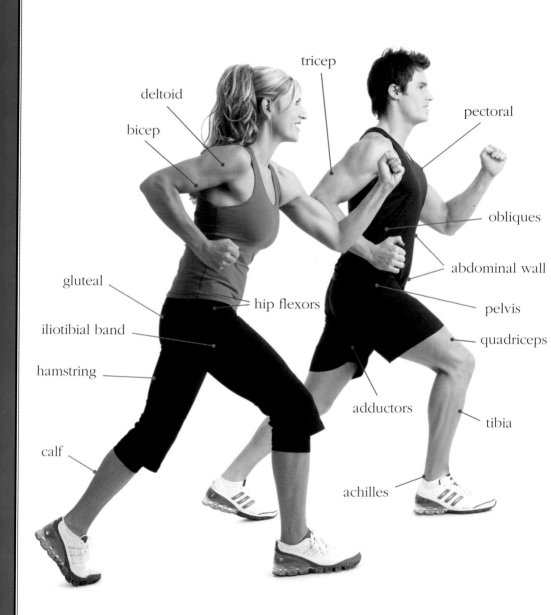

tricep

deltoid

pectoral

bicep

obliques

abdominal wall

gluteal

pelvis

hip flexors

iliotibial band

quadriceps

hamstring

adductors

tibia

calf

achilles

GLOSSARY

ABDOMINAL WALL
The entire sheet of muscle between the ribs and the hips.

ACHILLES
The thick tendon that connects the calf muscle to the heel bone.

ANTERIOR
Refers to the front of the body.

BODY COMPOSITION
The amount of body fat a person has in comparison to their total body mass.

BRACED CORE
The action of contracting the muscles in the abdominal wall.

CALVES
The muscles of the rear lower leg between the knee and ankle joint.

CARDIO
Relates to activity that elevates the heart rate.

DELTOIDS
The muscles that surround the shoulder joints.

DYNAMIC STRETCHING
Repeatedly taking a muscle to an elongated position with gentle recovery.

ELONGATE
To maintain a position of length and poise.

GAIT
A person's walking pattern.

GLUTEALS
The muscles of the buttocks, located at the base of the spine.

HAMSTRINGS
The muscles of the rear upper thigh, located between the hips and the knee joints.

HIP FLEXORS
The band of muscles in the front of the body, joining the torso to the thighs.

ILIOTIBIAL BAND
The lateral muscles of the hips, covering the outer hip joint.

LATERAL
Refers to the outer areas of the body.

OBLIQUES
The lateral muscles of the abdominal wall.

PECTORALS
The muscles of the upper body, covering the chest.

PELVIS
The bony structure at the base of the spine, incorporating the hip joints for each of the legs.

POSTERIOR
Refers to the back areas of the body.

QUADRICEPS
The muscles of the front upper thigh, located between the knee and hip joint.

REACTION TIME
The time it takes to react to stimuli.

RESPIRATORY
Relates to breathing or the lungs.

STATIC STRETCH
A stationary or fixed stretch.

SHOULDER BLADE (OR THE SCAPULA)
The two triangular bones located on either side of the upper back.

TORSO
The section of the body excluding the head, neck and limbs.

TRICEPS
The muscles of the rear upper arm, located between the elbow and shoulder joint.

CONCLUSION

To achieve success in your new fitness regime, you need motivation. Focus on the six 'P's to help you keep the motivation going. This creates habits: habits that you will repeat over and over without thinking, making them part of your lifestyle.

The six 'P's for a successful journey are:

PLAN
Making the decision to exercise is easy. Planning makes it easier to actually follow through. Know in advance what you'll need and have it ready for your workout. It can be as simple as leaving your workout gear beside the bed each night so when you wake, you associate starting the day with exercise. Prepare meals or snacks in advance and plan out what you'll do each day.

PRACTISE
A lot of our daily lives involves routines and habits. If you make exercise a habit, it becomes easier to do. Have a regular workout day and time so that once that time comes, you're ready to get busy! Create habits around your workout to help you get ready. For example, if you're a morning exerciser, take your vitamins with a glass of juice just prior to your workout. Find ways to make your workout a normal part of your life, just like brushing your teeth. Make exercise a necessity, not a luxury.

PROMISE
Being healthy isn't a decision you make once – it's one you make every day. Recommitting to your goals keeps you on track. Promise yourself you'll spend a few minutes each morning thinking or writing about what you want to accomplish that day and how you'll do it. Remind yourself of your goals and take time to appreciate how far you've come. Write them down and put them where you can see them. Do what you can to remind yourself of your commitment to exercise. Keep your promise!

PREPARE
Part of sticking to your routine is allowing some flexibility. Be prepared to change your routine. You may plan on jogging for 30 minutes, but don't have the time. Many of us would end up skipping our workout instead of coming up with an alternative. Have a plan in mind, but be prepared for unexpected changes. Always have a backup. If you have to work late, fit in a quick walk at lunch or use your breaks for some stair walking. It all counts!

Payment

Lack of motivation is the biggest barrier people face. We all want results now, although common sense tells us that results appear with perseverance and lifestyle changes. With perseverance comes payment, both external (improvement to your body shape) and internal (improved health). Remember to reward yourself for your efforts with another payment, it could be a massage at a local day spa or relaxation centre – but only if you finish your workouts!

Positive

All these words (plan, practise, promise, prepare, payment) don't sound like much fun. They sound like more work! Most of us have obligations and responsibilities that are work in themselves. Exercise often feels like just another duty. We forget that moving our bodies can actually be fun. Don't just try to find the time: make the time. This inevitably leads to a more positive experience and to a more positive you!

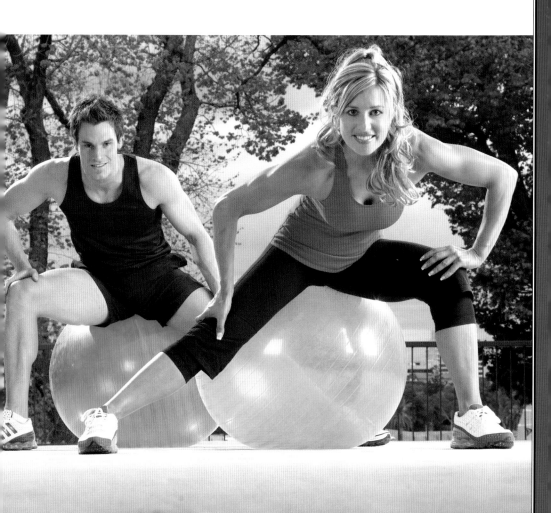

ABOUT THE AUTHOR

JULIA FILEP

Julia Filep has 17 years' experience in the fitness industry. Julia resides and works in Victoria, Australia, and is a specialist in many areas of group exercise delivery, instruction and communication. Her commitment to the industry is evident in the vast array of classes that she instructs and the high rate of long-term, regular participants that she maintains in those classes. Julia also trains other group exercise teachers and relishes the opportunity to pass on her experience and knowledge to others. Julia appeared in the personal fitness series *Heat* and has had more recent success with her book and DVD exercise program, *The Complete Ball and Web*. Julia is the mother of two young boys and she thrives on the challenge of balancing work and family life. Julia believes that more movement in our day creates quality longevity for all: a philosophy she wants to share with everyone.

GARETH DONALD

Gareth Donald is a personal trainer, strength and conditioning coach, and fitness and nutrition consultant. The proprietor of Shayah Fitness (which stands for strong, healthy and young at heart), Gareth provides unique and highly effective training, nutrition and supplementation programs for high level athletes as well as recreational exercisers.

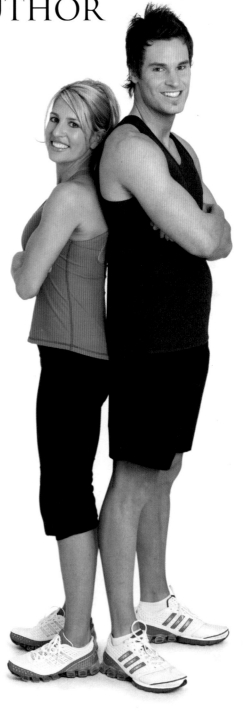